Copyright 2023

# Table of Contents

A stroke occurs when a blood vessel in the brain ruptures and bleeds, or when there's a blockage in the blood supply to the brain. The rupture or blockage prevents blood and oxygen from reaching the brain's tissues.

According to the Centers for Disease Control and Prevention (CDC) Trusted Source, stroke is a leading cause of death in the United States. Every year, more than 795,000 U.S. people have a stroke.

Without oxygen, brain cells and tissue become damaged and begin to die within minutes.

There are three primary types of strokes:

Transient ischemic attack (TIA) involves a blood clot that typically reverses on its own.

Ischemic stroke involves a blockage caused by either a clot or plaque in the artery. The symptoms and complications of ischemic stroke can last longer than those of a TIA, or may become permanent.

Hemorrhagic stroke is caused by either a burst or leaking blood vessel that seeps into the brain.

## BREAKFAST

### 1. Torrejas (Mexican French toast)

Prep Time: 15 Minutes

Cook Time: 20 Minutes

Servings: 8

Ingredients

For the piloncillo syrup:

- 16 ounces piloncillo
- 1 cinnamon stick
- 2 cloves
- 1 cup water

For the torrejas:

- 2 cups vegetable oil, for frying
- 6 large eggs
- 1 ½ cups milk
- ½ tablespoon vanilla extract

- 4 bolillo rolls, sliced into 16-18 slices about ¾ inches thick

Instructions

1. Make the piloncillo syrup: Add the piloncillo, cinnamon stick, cloves, and water into a medium saucepan. Cook over medium heat for 15 minutes, stirring occasionally, until the piloncillo fully melts and forms into a syrup. Remove from heat, carefully discard the cinnamon stick and cloves, and set aside until ready to serve.
2. Prepare the oil: Heat the frying oil in a large saucepan or deep skillet over medium-high heat. Line a baking sheet with paper towels and set aside. While oil is heating up, prepare the batter.
3. Make the batter: Separate the egg whites from the yolks into two separate bowls – the whites into a large mixing bowl and the yolks into a small bowl.
4. Using an electric hand mixer, beat the egg whites until stiff peaks form.
5. While continuing to beat the egg whites on low, add in the egg yolks one at a time until all of them are fully

mixed in. The batter should be light, fluffy, and smooth.

6. In a separate medium bowl, whisk together the milk and vanilla extract.

7. Coat the bread: Using tongs or your hands, dip a slice of bolillo bread into the milk mixture for 1-2 seconds, then gently tap it to remove any excess milk. Then dip it in the egg batter so that the bread is fully coated and gently place it in the frying oil.

8. Fry: Fry the torrejas for 30-45 seconds minutes per side, until the batter is golden brown and crispy. Try not to overcrowd the torrejas in the pan – I usually fry 3 at a time depending on the pan I'm using.

9. Serve: Serve the torrejas on a plate and drizzle with piloncillo syrup. Alternatively, you can also dip each of the torrejas into the syrup and serve coated in syrup.

Prep Time: 25 Minutes

Cook Time: 2hrs 5 Minutes

Servings: 10

Ingredients

For the chile sauce:

- 3 cups water
- 6 dried guajillo chiles, rinsed and seeds removed
- 4 dried ancho chiles, rinsed and seeds removed
- 2 dried arbol chiles, rinsed (seeds removed if you prefer a mild spice level)
- 1 ½ teaspoon coarse sea salt
- 3 teaspoons chili powder
- 2 teaspoons ground cumin
- 4 cloves garlic, minced
- 8 grams Mexican chocolate, optional (about ⅛ disc)

For the stew:

- 2 1/2 pounds pork shoulder, cut into large 4-inch chunks
- 1 tablespoon kosher salt

- 1 teaspoon black pepper
- 2 tablespoons oil
- 6 cups broth (chicken, vegetable, or beef)
- 3 (15-ounce) cans white hominy, drained and rinsed
- 1 tablespoon dried oregano (Mexican oregano preferred)
- Suggested toppings
- thinly shredded cabbage, cilantro, diced onions, lime wedges, sliced radishes, Mexican oregano, avocado

Instructions

1. Soak the chiles: In a small pot over high heat, bring the water to a boil. Remove it from the heat and add in the dried chiles. Cover and let the chiles soak for 10 minutes.
2. Blend the chiles: Carefully transfer the softened chiles and the hot water into a large blender. Add the salt, chili powder, ground cumin, garlic, and Mexican chocolate. Blend for 2-3 minutes until completely smooth. Set aside.
3. Prepare the meat: Season all sides of the pork with the salt and black pepper. Heat a large pot or Dutch oven over medium-high heat. Add in the cooking oil and

then the pork. Sear the meat on all sides until nicely browned.

4. Combine: Pour in the red chile sauce and scrape the bottom of the pot with a wooden spoon to loosen all the brown bits. Stir in the broth, hominy, and dried oregano.

5. Cook: Bring the pot to a boil, reduce heat to a low, cover and simmer for 2 ½ hours, until the pork is fall-apart tender.

6. Shred the meat: Shred the pork with a fork or tongs (it should fall apart very easily). Taste and season with more salt, if necessary.

7. Serve: Serve with toppings such as thinly shredded cabbage, cilantro, lime juice, sliced radishes, diced onions, avocados, and dried Mexican oregano.

Prep Time: 5 Minutes

Cook Time: 35 Minutes

Servings: 6


Ingredients

- 4 cups milk
- 2 ounces piloncillo, plus more to taste
- 2 (3-ounce) discs Mexican chocolate (I used Abuelita brand)
- 1 cinnamon stick
- 1 1/2 cups warm water
- 1/2 cup masa harina
- 2 teaspoons vanilla extract
- 1 pinch salt


Instructions

1. Add milk, piloncillo, Mexican chocolate, and cinnamon stick to a medium saucepan or pot. Heat over low-medium heat until the piloncillo and chocolate have

completely dissolved. Stir frequently to make sure nothing sticks to the bottom of the saucepan.

2. Remove and discard the cinnamon stick, using a strainer if it has broken into pieces.

3. In a small bowl, add warm water and masa harina. Whisk together until the mixture is smooth.

4. Add the masa harina mixture, vanilla extract, and salt to the saucepan. Whisk to combine.

5. Bring to a simmer, reduce heat to low, and continue to cook, whisking frequently, for 25-30 minutes until thick, creamy, velvety, and smooth. The champurrado should be thick enough to coat the back of a spoon.

6. Serve and garnish with a touch of ground cinnamon or a cinnamon stick.

Prep Time: 45 Minutes

Cook Time: 10 Minutes

Servings: 8


Ingredients

For the bunuelos:

- 2 cups all-purpose flour
- 1 1/2 teaspoon baking powder
- 1/2 teaspoon salt
- 3/4 cup warm water
- 4 tablespoons oil, plus 2 or more cups for frying

For the cinnamon sugar topping:

- 1/2 cup granulated sugar
- 1 tablespoon ground cinnamon


Instructions

For the bunuelos:

1. Add all-purpose flour, baking powder and salt in a large bowl. Mix together until combined.

2. Add warm water and 4 tablespoons oil. Mix together with a spoon or your hands until the dough comes together.

3. Transfer the dough onto a clean working surface and knead the dough for 8 to 10 minutes, until the dough is smooth and elastic.

4. Roll the dough into a ball, place it in a bowl, cover with a kitchen towel and let it rest for 30 minutes.

5. While the dough is resting, cover a large plate with paper towels, fill a large saute pan with 1 to 2 inches of frying oil and make the cinnamon sugar topping. Set aside.

6. Divide the dough into 8 separate pieces and roll each piece into a ball. On a lightly floured surface, use a floured rolling pin to roll out each ball into an 8 to 10-inch circle. (I recommend laying the rolled out dough onto a large kitchen towel in one single layer. Don't stack the rolled out dough on top of each other or it may stick.)

7. Heat the frying oil to 350°F. Fry each dough circle for about 60 seconds, turning once, until golden brown on both sides. Transfer to prepared plate to drain any

excess oil. Sprinkle heavily with cinnamon sugar topping.

8.  For the cinnamon sugar topping

9.  Combine granulated sugar and ground cinnamon in a small bowl.

Prep Time: 20 Minutes

Cook Time: 6hrs 3 Minutes

Servings: 6

Ingredients

- 2 tablespoon olive oil
- 1 large onion, diced
- 1 pound Honeysuckle White 93% Lean Ground Turkey
- 2 teaspoons coarse kosher salt, divided
- 2 cups chicken broth
- 1 15-ounce can fire-roasted diced tomatoes
- 1 15-ounce can black beans, drained and rinsed
- 1 15-ounce can pinto beans, drained and rinsed
- 1 15-ounce can whole corn kernels, drained and rinsed
- 2 tablespoons chili powder
- 1 teaspoon ground cumin
- 1 teaspoon smoked paprika
- 1/2 teaspoon dried oregano
- 2 tablespoons lime juice (about the juice of 1 lime)
- 1/4 cup chopped cilantro (optional)
- 4 ounces cream cheese (optional)

- optional toppings: tortilla strips and shredded cheese

Instructions

1. Heat olive oil in a large nonstick skillet over medium-high heat. Add onions and saute for 5 minutes until softened.

2. Add ground turkey and 1 teaspoon salt. Mix together and break up the meat using a spatula. Cook for 8-10 minutes, until the meat has browned and fully cooked through.

3. Transfer cooked ground turkey and onions to a large slow cooker. Add chicken broth, diced tomatoes, black beans, pinto beans, corn, the remaining 1 tablespoon salt, chili powder, and ground cumin, smoked paprika and dried oregano.

4. Mix together until fully combined. Cover and cook on low for 6-8 hours. The longer it cooks, the thicker and more concentrated the flavor of the broth will be.

5. Mix in lime juice, cilantro (if desired) and cream cheese (if you want the soup a little creamy).

6. Serve and top with tortilla strips and shredded cheese.

Prep Time: 5 Minutes

Cook Time: 4hrs 3 Minutes

Servings: 10


Ingredients

For the carnitas:

- 2 1/2 pounds pork shoulder (also known as 'pork butt')
- 1 tablespoon lime juice
- 2 teaspoons coarse sea salt
- 2 teaspoons ground cumin
- 1 teaspoon chili powder
- 1 teaspoon garlic powder
- 1 teaspoon dried oregano
- 1 teaspoon onion powder
- 1/2 teaspoon ground black pepper
- 1 cup broth (chicken, beef or vegetable) for Instant Pot cooking method only

Instructions

Slow Cooker Instructions:

1.  Cut the pork shoulder into large 4-inch chunks. Place in the slow cooker.
2.  Add the lime juice, salt, ground cumin, chili powder, garlic powder, dried oregano, onion powder and black pepper. Mix thoroughly to coat the meat with all the seasonings.
3.  Cover and cook on high for 4 hours, or on low for 7-8 hours. When tender, shred the meat by pulling it apart with two forks.
4.  Mix in freshly chopped cilantro if desired and serve in tacos, gorditas, tostadas, burrito bowls and salads.
5.  Instant Pot Instructions
6.  Cut the pork shoulder into large 4-inch chunks. Place in the Instant Pot.
7.  Add the lime juice, salt, ground cumin, chili powder, garlic powder, dried oregano, onion powder, black pepper and 1 cup of broth. Mix thoroughly to coat the meat with all the seasonings.
8.  Lock the lid and set the steam release vent to the "sealing" position. Press the "manual" button and set the timer on high pressure for 40 minutes.

9. When the 40 minutes are up, let the pressure naturally release for 15 minutes. Then manually release the remaining pressure by moving the steam release vent to the "venting" position.

10. Open the lid and shred the meat with two forks. Mix in freshly chopped cilantro if desired and serve in tacos, gorditas, tostadas, burrito bowls and salads.

Prep Time: 15 Minutes

Cook Time: 7hrs 3 Minutes

Servings: 7

Ingredients

- 1/2 pound dried lentils (about 1 cup + 2 tablespoons), green or brown
- 1 medium yellow onion, diced
- 2 medium carrots, diced
- 2 medium celery stalks, diced
- 2 teaspoons minced garlic (about 4 cloves)
- 1 chipotle pepper in adobo sauce + 1 tablespoon sauce, minced
- 1 teaspoon ground cumin
- 1/2 teaspoon coarse kosher salt, plus more to taste
- 1/2 teaspoon dried oregano
- 1 14-ounce can fire-roasted diced tomatoes
- 5 cups broth (vegetable or chicken)
- 1 bay leaf
- 2 tablespoons olive oil
- 2 teaspoons white wine vinegar

Instructions

1. Add all ingredients except the olive oil and white wine vinegar to the slow cooker. Cover and cook on low for 7-8 hours or on high for 5-6 hours, until the lentils are tender.

2. Discard the bay leaf and carefully ladle out about 4 cups of the soup into a large blender. Add the olive oil, cover and pulse a few times until semi-smooth and creamy looking.

3. Pour the blended soup into the crockpot and add the white wine vinegar. Stir to combine, taste and season with more salt to taste.

4. Serve with desired toppings like chopped cilantro, sour cream, shredded parmesan and crusty bread.

Prep Time: 10 Minutes

Cook Time: 8hrs 2 Minutes

Servings: 10

Ingredients

- 3 pounds boneless chuck roast
- salt and pepper, enough to coat meat
- 1 onion, quartered
- 2 teaspoons minced garlic (about 4 cloves)
- 1 bay leaf
- 4 chipotle peppers in adobo sauce, diced
- 1 teaspoon cumin
- 1 teaspoon oregano
- 1 tablespoon apple cider vinegar
- 1/4 cup water
- for serving: cilantro, red onions, tortillas and lime wedges

Instructions

1.  Cut the chuck roast into large chunks, removing any excess fat. Generously season all sides of the meat with sea salt and black pepper.
2.  Heat a large skillet over medium-high heat. Add the meat and sear on all sides.
3.  Place the meat and all other ingredients in a slow cooker. Mix together to coat the meat with all the herbs and spices.
4.  Cover and cook on low for 8 hours, or on high for 4-5 hours. When tender, shred the meat by pulling it apart with a fork. Taste and season with more salt as needed.
5.  Serve barbacoa in warm corn tortillas with chopped red onions, cilantro and lime juice.

Prep Time: 14 Minutes

Cook Time: 16 Minutes

Servings: 8


Ingredients

For the meat and quick marinade:

- 2 pounds boneless skinless chicken breast, sliced into thin strips
- 1/4 cup chopped cilantro
- 2 tablespoons lime juice (juice of 1 lime)
- 1 tablespoon cooking oil
- 1 tablespoon minced garlic (about 3 cloves)
- 1 tablespoon chili powder
- 1 teaspoon ground cumin
- 1 teaspoon dried oregano
- 1/2 teaspoon coarse kosher salt
- 1/2 teaspoon paprika
- 1/2 teaspoon ancho chili powder

For the peppers and onions

- 2 tablespoons cooking oil, divided

- 2 bell peppers, sliced into strips
- 1 large poblano pepper sliced into strips (or substitute with another bell pepper if you can't find poblanos)
- 1/2 large onion, sliced
- 1 pinch salt
- Optional toppings
- ▫guacamole, sour cream, chopped cilantro, flour or corn tortillas

Instructions

1. Add all the ingredients for the quick marinade in a large mixing bowl. Toss together until chicken is evenly coated with spices. Cover and set aside.
2. In a large skillet over medium-high heat, add 1 tablespoon of cooking oil. Add the peppers, onions and a pinch of salt. Cook, stirring occasionally, for about 8 minutes, until the veggies are soft.
3. Remove from the skillet, place in a large bowl, cover and set aside.
4. Add the remaining tablespoon of cooking oil to the same skillet. Add the marinated chicken and cook for 8 to 10 minutes, until chicken is fully cooked.

5.  Add the peppers and onions back to the skillet, toss together with the chicken and remove from heat.

6.  Serve in warm flour or corn tortillas and top with sour cream, guacamole and chopped cilantro.

Prep Time: 5 Minutes

Cook Time: 25 Minutes

Servings: 6

Ingredients

- 3 tablespoons olive oil
- 1 medium onion, diced
- 1 jalapeno, seeds and stem removed (optional)
- 1 teaspoon minced garlic (about 2 cloves)
- 1/2 cup masa harina
- 3 cups chicken broth
- 2 1/4 cups red enchilada sauce (authentic version, easy 10-minute version, or 2 10-ounce cans)
- 3 cups cooked shredded chicken (about 1 1/2 pounds)
- 1 14-ounce can black beans, rinsed and drained
- 1 14-ounce can fire-roasted diced tomatoes
- 2 4-ounce cans green chiles
- 1 teaspoon salt, plus more to taste
- 4 ounces cream cheese

Instructions

1. Heat olive oil in a large Dutch oven or pot over medium-high heat. Add onions, jalapeno (if using) and garlic and saute for 5 minutes, until onions become translucent.

2. Add masa harina and cook for 1 minute, stirring constantly.

3. Add chicken broth, enchilada sauce, shredded chicken, black beans, diced tomatoes, green chiles and salt.

4. Stir together to combine and cook for about 10 minutes, uncovered, until the soup begins to simmer. Make sure to stir the soup occasionally to make sure the masa harina gets fully distributed throughout the soup.

5. Remove the Dutch oven or pot from the heat and add the cream cheese. Stir it into the soup until it completely dissolves and melts.

6. Serve immediately with your favorite toppings and enjoy!

## 11. Molletes

Prep Time: 10 Minutes

Cook Time: 5 Minutes

Servings: 4

Ingredients

- 2 bolillo bread rolls (homemade or store bought)
- 2 tablespoons butter or margarine
- 1 cup refried beans (homemade or store bought)
- 1 cup Monterey Jack shredded cheese
- 1/2 cup pico de gallo or your favorite Mexican salsa

Instructions

1. Line a large baking sheet with parchment paper and set aside.
2. Slice bolillo bread rolls in half lengthwise. Spread 1/2 tablespoon of butter on each slice.
3. Place rolls on prepared baking sheet buttered side up and put in oven on the middle rack.

4. Broil for 2-3 minutes, until lightly toasted.

5. Remove from oven and top each slice with a layer of 1/4 cup refried beans and 1/4 cup shredded cheese.

6. Place molletes in oven one more time and broil for 3-4 minutes, until cheese has melted and is bubbly. Make sure to keep an eye on it during this time as the bread can quickly start to burn.

7. Top each slice with 2 tablespoons of pico de gallo. Serve immediately.

Prep Time: 10 Minutes

Cook Time: 20 Minutes

Servings: 8


Ingredients

- 2 small-medium gold potatoes, diced (about 2 cups)
- 1 16-ounce bag frozen mixed vegetables
- 4 cups cooked shredded chicken (about 1 lb cooked)
- 3/4 cup mayonnaise
- 1/4 cup sour cream
- juice of 1 lime (about 2 tablespoons)
- 1 tablespoon brine from pickled jalapenos, mild or hot (optional)
- 3/4 teaspoon coarse kosher salt, plus more to taste


Instructions

1. In a small saucepan, add potatoes. Cover completely with water, cover with lid, and bring to a boil over high heat.

2. Reduce heat to simmer and cook for 8 minutes, or until potatoes are cooked through. Carefully drain the water and set aside.

3. In a medium microwave-safe bowl, add the frozen mixed vegetables and microwave on high for 4-6 minutes, stirring halfway through, until fully thawed. Set aside.

4. In a small bowl, add the mayonnaise, sour cream, lime juice, pickled jalapeno brine, and salt. Whisk together to combine.

5. In a large bowl, add the cooked potatoes, thawed mixed vegetables, shredded chicken, and mayonnaise mixture. Toss together to combine.

6. Taste and season with more salt or pickled jalapeno brine to your liking.

7. Refrigerate for 1-2 hours, or until chilled. Serve with saltine crackers, on tostada shells, with tortilla chips, or in a sandwich.

Prep Time: 5 Minutes

Cook Time: 15 Minutes

Servings: 10


Ingredients

For the fruit salsa:

- 1 pound strawberries, diced
- 1/2 pound grapes, halved
- 2 large oranges, diced
- 4 kiwis, diced
- 1 red apple, diced
- 1 pint blueberries
- 1 lemon, for juicing (or 3 tablespoons lemon juice)

For the cinnamon chips:

- cooking spray
- 1/3 cup granulated sugar
- 1 tablespoon ground cinnamon
- 10 medium (soft taco size) flour tortillas

Instructions

For the fruit salsa:

1. In a large bowl, add all the ingredients. Toss together to combine and serve immediately or cover and chill in the fridge until ready to eat.
2. For the cinnamon chips
3. Preheat oven to 350°F. Spray two large baking sheets with cooking spray.
4. In a small bowl, add sugar and cinnamon. Mix together until fully combined.
5. Cut flour tortillas into 8 triangles each (like you would cut a pizza) for a total of 80 triangles.
6. Place the tortilla triangles onto the prepared baking sheets in one single layer, making sure they don't overlap with any others. You may have to bake them in two or three batches, depending on the size of your baking sheets.
7. Spray the tortillas with cooking spray and sprinkle with cinnamon sugar. Flip them over and do this again on the other side. Bake for 15 minutes, until golden brown and crispy.

Prep Time: 10 Minutes

Cook Time: 2hr 35 Minutes

Servings: 12

Ingredients

- 1 pound dried pinto beans (see tips below for using canned beans)
- water
- 1/2 pound uncooked bacon
- 1 small onion, diced
- 1 jalapeno, diced (seeds and veins removed if you don't want it spicy)
- 4 cloves garlic, minced
- 2 teaspoons chili powder
- 1 teaspoon ancho chili powder (or regular if you don't have ancho)
- 1 teaspoon dried oregano (Mexican oregano preferred)
- 1 teaspoon coarse kosher salt
- 1/2 teaspoon ground cumin
- 1 14-ounce can diced tomatoes

- 1 12-ounce bottle dark lager beer (I used Negra Modelo)
- 1 tablespoon dark brown sugar
- 1/4 cup chopped cilantro

Instructions

1. Pour the beans into a large bowl. Pick out and discard any beans that are shriveled or split as well as any small rocks that may have made their way into the bag.
2. Fully cover the beans with water (at least 3 inches over the top of the beans) and set on the counter to soak for 8 hours or overnight.
3. Drain and rinse the beans under cool water. (They will have doubled in size during the soaking process!)
4. Transfer the beans to a large pot or Dutch oven. Add 10 cups of water (and the optional ingredients if using them).
5. Bring beans to a boil, then reduce heat to a low simmer. Cover and cook for 2 to 2 1/2 hours. (I recommend checking them at the 2 hour mark and giving them a taste. They should be tender and fully cooked through, but still a little firm and not mushy. Cook a little longer if they're not quite done.)

6. Drain cooked beans, transfer to a large bowl, and set aside. Rinse and dry the pot.

7. Return pot to the stove and heat over medium-high heat. Add the bacon and cook, stirring occasionally, until browned and crispy. Transfer the cooked bacon to a plate lined with paper towels and set aside.

8. Add the onions and jalapeno and cook for 5 minutes, scraping up any browned bits on the bottom of the pot.

9. Add the garlic, chili powders, dried oregano, salt and ground cumin. Stir and cook for 30 seconds.

10. Add the cooked pinto beans, diced tomatoes, beer and brown sugar. Stir together to combine and bring to a low simmer.

11. Simmer the beans for 15 minutes and remove from heat. Stir in the chopped cilantro and crispy bacon. Serve immediately.

Prep Time: 15 Minutes

Cook Time: 1hr 35 Minutes

Servings: 6

Ingredients

For the red chile sauce:

- 8 dried Guajillo chiles, stems removed and seeded
- 2 dried Ancho chiles, stems removed and seeded
- 1 dried Arbol chile, stem removed and seeded (or more if you like spicy food)
- 1/2 medium yellow onion, quartered
- 1 teaspoon dried oregano
- 1 teaspoon salt
- 1 clove garlic
- 1/2 teaspoon cumin

For the meat:

- 2 pounds beef stew meat (like chuck shoulder or roast), cut into 1/2 inch squares
- 2 tablespoons all purpose flour
- 1/2 teaspoon salt, plus more to taste

- 1/4 teaspoon black pepper
- 2 tablespoons cooking oil
- 3 cups beef broth, divided (or chicken or vegetable broth)
- 2 bay leaves

Instructions

For the red chile sauce:

1. In a medium pot, add dried Guajillo chiles, Ancho chiles, Arbol chiles, and onion to a medium pot. Cover with water until chiles and onions are completely submerged and bring to a boil over high heat. Once boiling, remove from heat, cover and let it sit for 20 minute to soften the peppers.
2. Using a slotted spoon, transfer the softened chiles and onions into a large blender. Add in 1 cup of the chile-soaked water, the dried oregano, salt, garlic and cumin. Blend until smooth. Add some of the beef broth from the meat ingredients as needed if the mixture is too thick for your blender.
3. Once the red chile sauce is as smooth as possible, pour it through a strainer into a bowl, pushing down on the

solids that accumulate to get as much moisture out as possible. Discard the solids.

For the meat:

1. In a large bowl, add the beef, flour, salt and pepper. Toss together to coat.
2. Heat a large pot or dutch oven, heat the oil over medium-high heat. Add in half of the meat and brown on all sides so they have a good sear, about 5 minutes. Transfer the browned beef into a bowl and repeat the process with the remaining uncooked meat.
3. Once the second batch of meat has browned, return all the meat into the pot. Add in the red chile sauce, beef broth and bay leaves. Stir to combine and bring to boil. Once boiling, reduce heat to simmer, cover and cook for 45 minutes.
4. Uncover, taste and add more salt as necessary. Raise to medium heat and cook for another 15 to 30 minutes, until the sauce has reduced and thickened slightly. If you prefer a thicker sauce, cook longer.
5. Discard bay leaves and serve with Mexican rice and beans.

Prep Time: 20 Minutes

Cook Time: 00 Minutes

Servings: 6

## Ingredients

- 1/4 medium-large watermelon, peeled and cubed (about 4 cups)
- 1 pineapple, peeled, cored and cubed (about 4 cups)
- 2 mangoes, peeled, seeded and cubed (about 2 cups)
- 1 jicama, peeled and cubed (about 2 cups)
- Tajin seasoning, for topping to taste (I recommend about 1/2 teaspoon per cup)
- chamoy sauce, for topping to taste (I recommend about 1 tablespoon per cup)
- lime wedges, for topping plus more to taste

## Instructions

1. Evenly distribute the fruit into 6 18-ounce clear plastic cups or 12 9-ounce clear plastic cups.

2.  Top each fruit cup with a sprinkle of Tajin seasoning, a drizzle of chamoy sauce and a lime wedge.

3.  Place a fork in each cup and serve immediately.

Prep Time: 10 Minutes

Cook Time: 00 Minutes

Servings: 6

Ingredients

- 1 pound fresh strawberries
- 2 cups sour cream
- 1 cup sweetened condensed milk
- 1/2 cup evaporated milk
- 1/2 teaspoon vanilla extract

Instructions

1. Remove and discard the stems from the strawberries. Slice the fruit into thin slices and transfer to a medium bowl.
2. In a large mixing bowl, add sour cream, sweetened condensed milk, evaporated milk and vanilla extract. Whisk together to combine.
3. Scoop 1/2 cup sliced strawberries into 6 bowls or cups. Then top each cup with 1/2 cup sweet cream mixture.

4.  Serve immediately with a spoon or store in the fridge
    for up to 5 days.

Prep Time: 1hr 5 Minutes

Cook Time: 25 Minutes

Servings: 18


Ingredients

For the dough:

- 3 ¾ cups all-purpose flour
- ¾ teaspoon fine salt
- ¾ cup cold unsalted butter, cut into ½-inch cubes
- 2 large eggs, chilled and divided
- ¾ cup ice water

For the filling:

- 1 tablespoon oil
- 1 plum tomato, diced
- ¼ medium yellow onion, diced
- 2 cloves garlic, minced
- 1 pound lean ground beef
- 1 teaspoon chili powder
- 1 teaspoon kosher salt
- ½ teaspoon ground cumin

- ¼ teaspoon dried oregano
- ¼ teaspoon ground coriander
- 1 small russet potato, diced
- 1 medium carrot, diced
- ½ cup beef broth (or water)
- ¼ cup frozen peas
- 1 cup shredded cheddar cheese

Instructions

1. Make the pastry dough: In a food processor, add the all-purpose flour and salt. Pulse to combine. Add the butter, 1 egg, and ice water. Pulse until the mixture resembles coarse crumbs. (You may need to do this in batches depending on the size of your food processor.)

2. Transfer the dough mixture onto a clean surface and knead it for 5 minutes until it comes together and is smooth. Shape it into 2 equal sized balls, tightly cover each in plastic wrap, and refrigerate while you make the filling.

3. Make the filling: In a large skillet over medium-high heat, add the oil. When hot, add the tomato and onion, and cook for 5 minutes, stirring occasionally. Add the garlic and cook for 30 seconds, until fragrant.

4.  Add the ground beef, chili powder, salt, ground cumin, dried oregano, and ground coriander, and cook for 6-8 minutes, using a spoon to break up the meat into smaller pieces and stirring occasionally.

5.  Stir in the potato, carrot, and water, then reduce the heat to medium-low, cover, and cook for 10 minutes until the potatoes and carrots are soft and tender.

6.  Remove the skillet from heat, taste, and season with more salt if desired. Stir in the frozen peas and set aside.

7.  Remove the dough balls from the refrigerator and divide them into 18 equal pieces, then roll each piece into a ball.

8.  On a lightly floured surface, roll each ball evenly into a 6½ -7-inch circle with a rolling pin.

9.  In a small bowl, beat the remaining egg with a fork to make an egg wash.

10. Working one at a time, add 3-4 tablespoons of filling to one side of the empanada round and top with a small pinch of shredded cheese.

11. Using a pastry brush, brush the inside edge of the empanada round, then fold the dough in half over the filling.

12. Seal the empanada by pressing the edges together with the tines of a fork or folding over the edges in increments with your fingers. Repeat until all the empanadas are filled and sealed.

13. Transfer the empanadas to 2 large baking sheets lined with parchment paper, and refrigerate for 15 minutes.

14. Preheat the oven to 400°F with the rack in the center of the oven.

15. Brush the tops of each empanada with the remaining egg wash and bake for 25-30 min or until golden brown. Let them cool for 10 minutes before serving.

Prep Time: 10 Minutes

Cook Time: 20 Minutes

Servings: 8

Ingredients

- 1 cup yellow cornmeal
- 1 cup all-purpose flour
- ¼ cup granulated sugar
- 1 tablespoon baking powder
- ¼ teaspoon kosher salt
- 1 cup milk
- 2 large eggs
- 4 tablespoons unsalted butter, melted
- ½ cup cream-style corn
- ¼ cup shredded sharp cheddar cheese
- 2 large jalapeno peppers, finely diced
- 1 tablespoon oil or butter

Instructions

1. Place a 9 or 10-inch cast iron skillet on the middle rack in the oven, and preheat to 400°F.
2. In a large bowl, whisk together the cornmeal, flour, sugar, baking powder, and salt.
3. In a medium bowl, whisk together the milk, eggs, butter, and cream-style corn.
4. Add the wet ingredients to the dry ingredients and stir together until well combined. Fold in the shredded cheese and jalapenos until just combined.
5. Carefully remove the hot cast iron skillet form the oven and add the oil or butter to grease the skillet.
6. Pour the batter into the skillet, and bake for 20-25 minutes, until lightly browned and a toothpick inserted in the center comes out clean. Let cool for 10 minutes before serving.

Prep Time: 5 Minutes

Cook Time: 25 Minutes

Servings: 8

Ingredients

- 2 cups long grain white rice
- ¼ cup oil (vegetable or canola oil)
- ½ medium onion, finely diced
- 1 roma tomato, diced
- 4 cloves garlic, minced
- 1 ½ teaspoons kosher salt, plus more to taste
- 3 ½ cups broth (vegetable or chicken)
- 2 tablespoons tomato paste
- ½ cup frozen peas

Instructions

1. Add rice to a fine mesh strainer or colander and rinse under running water until the water runs clear. Drain well.

2. In a large saucepan or pot over low-medium heat, add the oil. When hot, add the rice and saute for 10 minutes, stirring frequently, until the rice begins to lightly brown.

3. Add the onion, tomato, garlic and salt. Stir and saute for 30 seconds.

4. Add the broth and tomato paste. Stir together to mix until the tomato paste has completely dissolved.

5. Bring to a boil, reduce heat to low, cover, and let cook for 20 minutes. Remove the saucepan or pot from the heat, uncover, and let it sit for 5 minutes.

6. Add the frozen peas and gently fluff the rice with a fork. Don't stir it. Taste and season with more salt if necessary.

Prep Time: 15 Minutes

Cook Time: 1hr 15 Minutes

Servings: 10

Ingredients

- 3-4 pounds boneless beef chuck roast
- kosher salt, enough to generously coat meat
- coarsely ground black pepper, enough to generously coat meat
- 2 ½ tablespoons oil, divided
- 1 medium onion, diced
- 6 cloves garlic, minced
- 1 cup beer, broth, or water
- 1/4 cup apple cider vinegar
- 1 lime, juiced
- 4 chipotle peppers in adobo sauce, diced
- 1 tablespoon ancho chili powder* (or regular chili powder)
- 1 tablespoon regular chili powder

- 2 teaspoons ground cumin

- 1 teaspoon dried oregano (Mexican oregano preferred)

- 1/4 teaspoon ground cloves

- 2 bay leaves

- for serving: chopped cilantro, diced onions, warm tortillas, and lime wedges

## Instructions

1. Cut the beef chuck roast into large 4-inch chunks, removing any large pieces of fat. Generously season all sides of the meat with salt and black pepper.

2. Press the saute button on the pressure cooker. When hot, add 1 1/2 tablespoons of oil and 3 or 4 pieces of meat. Brown the meat on all sides, flipping every 60 seconds. When browned, transfer to a plate and set aside. Continue working in batches until all the meat is browned.

3. Add the remaining 1 tablespoon of oil and the onions. Cook for 5 minutes, stirring often, making sure to scrape up any brown bits on the bottom of the pot.

4. Add the garlic and cook for 1 minute.

5. Add the beer (or broth or water), apple cider vinegar, lime juice, chipotle peppers in adobo sauce, ancho chili

powder, chili powder, ground cumin, dried oregano, ground cloves, and bay leaves. Stir together to combine.

6. Add in the seared meat and toss with the liquid to combine.
7. Close the lid of the pressure cooker and move the valve to the sealing position. Press the Manual or Pressure Cook button to high pressure, then adjust the +/- buttons until the time reads 60 minutes.
8. Let the pressure release naturally for 10 minutes, then release the remaining pressure carefully moving the venting position.
9. Remove the lid and shred the meat by pulling it apart with two fork. Taste and season with more salt as needed.
10. Serve barbacoa in warm corn tortillas with chopped onions, cilantro and lime juice, or on the side with rice and beans.

Prep Time: 40 Minutes

Cook Time: 15 Minutes

Servings: 8


Ingredients

For the marinade:

- 4 tablespoons olive oil
- 2 teaspoons white wine vinegar
- 2 teaspoons chili powder
- 2 teaspoons ancho chili powder*
- 1 1/2 teaspoon salt
- 1 teaspoon onion powder
- 1 teaspoon garlic powder
- 1/2 teaspoon ground cumin
- 1/2 teaspoon smoked paprika
- 1/2 teaspoon coarse ground black pepper
- 2 limes, juiced (about 4 tablespoons)

For the tacos:

- 2 pounds boneless skinless chicken thighs
- 24 corn tortillas (or flour tortillas)

- pico de gallo or your favorite salsa (optional)
- queso fresco or your favorite cheese (optional)

Instructions

1. In a large bowl, baking dish or freezer bag, add all the ingredients for the marinade. Mix together to fully combine.
2. Add chicken thighs to marinade and toss together to coat. Cover chicken and refrigerate for 30 minutes.
3. Heat a large non-stick skillet over medium-high heat. Add the marinated chicken to the skillet with tongs and cook 5-7 minutes per side, until fully cooked through. Discard the used marinade.
4. Transfer chicken to cutting board and let rest for 5 minutes. While chicken is resting, warm up the corn tortillas on a hot griddle or in the microwave.
5. Cut the chicken into bite-sized chunks and serve in warm tortillas with salsa and cheese.

Prep Time: 7 Minutes

Cook Time: 21 Minutes

Servings: 14

## Ingredients

- 2 cups cooked shredded chicken
- ½ tablespoon chili powder
- ½ teaspoon garlic powder
- ½ teaspoon ground cumin
- ½ teaspoon onion powder
- salt, to taste
- 1 ½ cups shredded cheese (Monterey Jack or Mexican blend)
- 14 corn tortillas
- cooking spray

## Instructions

1. In a medium bowl, add the shredded chicken, chili powder, garlic powder, ground cumin, onion powder

and salt in a bowl. Toss together to combine. Taste and season with more salt if necessary.

2.  Wrap the tortillas in a damp paper towel and heat them in the microwave for 1-2 minutes, flipping the tortillas halfway through until all of them are warm and pliable.

3.  Place a heaping spoonful of shredded chicken and shredded cheese onto each tortilla. Tightly roll up the tortillas and secure it closed by threading a toothpick along the seam (see photo in blog post).

4.  Preheat air fryer to 400°F. Place the taquitos in a single layer in the basket of the air fryer seam side down. Depending on how big your air fryer is, you will likely have to cook in multiple batches. Spray the taquitos with cooking spray, air fry for 5 minutes, flip and spray again, then air fry for 2 more minutes. Transfer to a plate and repeat with remaining taquitos.

5.  Remove the toothpicks from the taquitos and serve with shredded lettuce, pico de gallo, mexican crema and guacamole.

Prep Time: 10 Minutes

Cook Time: 12 Minutes

Servings: 4

## Ingredients

- 6 tablespoons unsalted butter
- 1/4 medium onion, thinly sliced
- 1/2 teaspoon kosher salt
- 1/4 teaspoon ground black pepper
- 6 cloves garlic, minced
- 1 lime, zested
- 1/2 lime, juiced
- 1 pound jumbo shrimp, peeled and deveined
- 1/2 teaspoon chopped cilantro

## Instructions

1. Heat the butter in a large skillet over medium heat until it fully melts.
2. Add the onion, salt, and black pepper. Cook for 2 minutes, stirring occasionally.

3.  Add the garlic and cook for 3 more minutes, stirring frequently until the garlic is fragrant and the onion becomes translucent.

4.  Add the lime zest and lime juice. Cook for 2 more minutes, stirring occasionally.

5.  Raise the heat to medium-high and add the shrimp. Cook for 3-4 minutes, flipping the shrimp halfway through, until the shrimp turns pink and is just cooked.

6.  Remove from heat, garnish with cilantro, and serve immediately.

Prep Time: 5 Minutes

Cook Time: 8 Minutes

Servings: 6

Ingredients

- 1/2 cup orange juice
- 1/4 cup lime juice (about 2 limes)
- 1/4 cup olive oil
- 2 tablespoons soy sauce
- 2 tablespoons Worcestershire sauce
- 1 tablespoon apple cider vinegar
- 3 cloves garlic, minced
- 1/2 teaspoon crushed red pepper flakes
- 1/4 teaspoon ground cumin
- 1 1/2 pounds skirt steak
- 1 teaspoon kosher salt
- 1/2 teaspoon coarse ground black pepper

Instructions

1. In a medium bowl, add the orange juice, lime juice, olive oil, soy sauce, Worcestershire sauce, apple cider vinegar, garlic, red pepper flakes, and ground cumin. Whisk together to combine.

2. Place the skirt steak in a large baking dish or gallon size zip-top bag and pour the marinade on top. Turn the steak a few times until it's completely coated with marinade, cover, and refrigerate for 2 to 6 hours. Do not marinate for longer than 8 hours because the meat will start to break down.

3. Remove steak from marinade and discard any excess marinade. Pat steak dry with paper towels and season with salt and black pepper on both sides.

4. To grill: Preheat grill to high heat (about 450°F-500°F). Grill the skirt steak with the lid closed for about 3-4 minutes per side for medium rare, or longer depending on the thickness and your desired doneness. I recommend using an instant-read meat thermometer to make sure it's perfect!

5. To cook on the stove: Heat a large cast-iron skillet over high heat with a generous drizzle of oil. Add the skirt steak and press down on the meat a couple of times to make sure it's fully touching the bottom of the pan (you

want to get a good sear). Cook for 3-5 minutes, then flip and cook for another 3-5 minutes depending on the thickness and your desired doneness. I recommend using an instant-read meat thermometer to make sure it's perfect!

6. Transfer the steak to a cutting board and let it rest for 5 minutes. Slice thinly across the grain and at a slight angle and serve.

Prep Time: 10 Minutes

Cook Time: 25 Minutes

Servings: 6

Ingredients

- 2 tablespoons Mazola Corn Oil
- 1/2 yellow onion, diced
- 2 cloves garlic, minced
- 1 1/2 pounds boneless skinless chicken breast, cut into 1-inch chunks
- 1 tablespoon chili powder
- 1/2 tablespoon kosher salt
- 1/2 tablespoon ground cumin
- 1 teaspoon smoked paprika
- 1 yellow squash, quartered and sliced into ½-inch pieces
- 1 zucchini, quartered and sliced into ½-inch pieces
- 1 cup fresh whole kernel corn, sliced off from 2 medium ears of corn
- 2 roma tomatoes, quartered
- 1/2 cup shredded cheddar cheese

- chopped cilantro, for garnish

- lime wedges, for garnish

## Instructions

1. Heat Mazola Corn Oil in a large skillet over medium-high heat. Add onion and garlic. Saute for 3 minutes.

2. Add chicken, chili powder, salt, cumin, and smoked paprika. Cook for 6-8 minutes, stirring occasionally, until chicken is cooked through.

3. Add yellow squash, zucchini, corn, and tomatoes. Cook for 8-10 minutes, stirring occasionally, until squash starts to become tender.

4. Remove from heat, top with shredded cheese, cover, and let sit for 3-5 minutes, until the cheese completely melts.

5. Garnish with chopped cilantro and limes wedges.

Prep Time: 10 Minutes

Cook Time: 30 Minutes

Servings: 4

Ingredients

- 4 medium russet potatoes, scrubbed and rinsed
- 1 1/2 tablespoons Mazola Corn Oil, divided
- 1 teaspoon kosher salt, divided
- 3/4 teaspoon garlic powder, divided
- 1/2 teaspoon onion powder
- 1/2 pound ground turkey (or chicken or beef)
- 1/4 teaspoon smoked paprika
- 1/4 teaspoon chili powder
- 1/4 teaspoon black pepper
- 1 1/4 cup shredded cheese (cheddar, monterey jack, or mozzarella)

Topping suggestions:

- diced red onions
- diced tomatoes
- chopped cilantro

- sour cream

- guacamole

## Instructions

1. Preheat oven to 450°F. Line a large baking sheet with parchment paper and set aside.

2. Cut potatoes into wedges by slicing each potato in half lengthwise, then slicing each of those halves in half again, and slicing those halves in half one last time. Each potato should yield 8 wedges.

3. Add potato wedges to a medium bowl and add 1 tablespoon Mazola® Corn Oil, 1/2 tablespoon kosher salt, 1/2 teaspoon garlic powder, and 1/2 teaspoon onion powder. Toss together to coat.

4. Place the wedges in a single layer on the prepared baking sheet. Bake for 25 minutes, flipping halfway through. While the potatoes are baking, prepare the ground turkey.

5. Heat remaining 1/2 tablespoon Mazola® Corn Oil in a large skillet over medium-high heat. Add ground chicken, the remaining 1/2 tablespoon kosher salt, the remaining 1/4 teaspoon garlic powder, 1/4 teaspoon

smoked paprika, 1/4 teaspoon chili powder, and 1/4 teaspoon black pepper.

6. Cook for 8-10 minutes, stirring occasionally, until the chicken is completely cooked. Set aside until ready to use.

7. When the potato wedges are finished, remove them from the oven. Push the potatoes together into a pile in the middle of the baking sheet. Top with the cooked seasoned ground turkey and the shredded cheese.

8. Return to the oven and bake for 3-5 minutes, until the cheese completely melts.

9. Top with diced onions, chopped cilantro, diced tomatoes, sour cream, and any other nacho toppings you like. Serve immediately.

Prep Time: 10 Minutes

Cook Time: 32 Minutes

Servings: 8


## Ingredients

- 1 tablespoon olive oil
- 1 medium onion, diced
- 1 jalapeño, stem and seeds removed, minced
- 1 pound lean ground beef
- 2 cloves garlic, minced
- 1 teaspoon coarse kosher salt, plus more to taste
- 1 3/4 cups easy enchilada sauce, divided
- 8 large flour tortillas
- 2 cups shredded Mexican-blend cheese, divided
- optional toppings: diced onions, chopped cilantro, sour cream, shredded lettuce


## Instructions

1. Preheat oven to 350°F.

2.  Heat olive oil in a large skillet over medium-high heat. Add the onions and jalapeño. Saute for 5 minutes, stirring occasionally, until softened and translucent.

3.  Add the ground beef, garlic, and salt. Use a wooden spoon to break up the meat into smaller chunks. Cook, stirring occasionally, for 6 to 8 minutes, until beef is browned.

4.  Add 1/4 cup enchilada sauce, stir to combine, and remove from heat. Taste and season with more salt if necessary.

5.  Microwave the tortillas on a plate for 1 minute, flipping them halfway through until all of them are warm and pliable.

6.  Pour 1/4 cup of the enchilada sauce into a 9×13 baking dish, and spread it out to fully coat the bottom.

7.  Assemble the enchiladas by filling each tortilla evenly with the beef mixture and 3/4 cup of shredded cheese. Roll the tortillas tightly to close and place in a large baking dish seam side down.

8.  Pour the remaining 1 1/4 cups enchilada sauce over the tortillas, top with the remaining 1 1/4 cups shredded cheese, and bake for 20 minutes, until the cheese is melted and bubbly.

Serve immediately and garnish with desired toppings.

Prep Time: 15 Minutes

Cook Time: 40 Minutes

Servings: 8

Ingredients

- 2 tablespoons olive oil
- 1 medium onion, diced
- 1 bell pepper, diced
- 2 cloves garlic, minced
- 1 cup cooked black beans
- 1 cup cooked yellow corn
- 3 cups cooked shredded chicken
- 1 (4-ounce) can diced green chilis
- 2 1/4 cups red enchilada sauce, divided
- 15 corn tortillas
- 3 1/2 cups shredded cheese, divided
- optional toppings: sour cream, chopped cilantro, diced avocado

Instructions

1.  Preheat oven to 350°F.
2.  Heat olive oil in a large skillet over medium heat. Add onion and pepper. Cook for 5 minutes, until softened.
3.  Add garlic and cook for 30 seconds, until fragrant.
4.  Add black beans, corn, shredded chicken, and green chilis. Cook for 5 minutes until warmed through. Remove from heat.
5.  Spread 1/2 cup enchilada sauce into the bottom of a 9×13 baking dish.
6.  Layer 5 tortillas into the dish so that it completely covers the bottom. Spread 1/3 of the chicken filling over tortillas, then top with 1/2 cup enchilada sauce and 1 cup of shredded cheese.
7.  Repeat 2 more times. On the last and final layer, top with all the remaining enchilada sauce and shredded cheese.
8.  Bake for 30 minutes, or until the cheese has melted and the sauce is bubbling.
9.  Garnish with sour cream, cilantro, and avocado.

Prep Time: 10 Minutes

Cook Time: 50 Minutes

Servings: 10

Ingredients

- oil or butter, for greasing
- 4 large bolillo bread rolls, cut into 1-inch thick pieces (about 10-12 cups)
- 5 cups nonfat milk
- 1 (8-ounce) cone piloncillo (or 1 1/4 cup dark brown sugar)
- 3 cinnamon sticks
- 2 whole cloves
- 3 large bananas, sliced into rounds
- 1 cup raisins
- 1/2 cup sliced almonds
- 2 cups shredded Oaxaca cheese (or any melty white cheese like Monterey Jack, Provolone or Mozzarella)

Instructions

1.  Preheat the oven to 350°F. Grease a 9×13-inch baking dish (or a dish that's slightly bigger) with oil or butter. Set aside.

2.  Place the cubed bolillo bread onto a large baking sheet. Bake it for 5 minutes so that bread become a little toasted and dried out. Remove it from oven and set aside.

3.  Add the milk, piloncillo, cinnamon sticks, and cloves to a large pot over medium-high heat. Whisk it together and bring it to a gentle boil.

4.  Reduce the heat to low and simmer it for 10 minutes, uncovered, whisking occasionally. Remove it from the heat and discard the cinnamon sticks and cloves.

5.  Assemble the capirotada by spreading half of the toasted bread in a single layer in the prepared baking dish. Top it with all of the banana slices, half of the raisins, half of the sliced almonds and half of the shredded cheese. Repeat the process with the remaining ingredients to make one more layer.

6.  Carefully pour the sweetened milk all over the capirotada, paying close attention to the bread on the edges.

7. Cover the dish with aluminum foil and bake for another 15 minutes, then remove the foil and bake it uncovered for 15 more minutes.

8. Remove it from the oven, let it cool for 5 minutes, and serve warm. Or let it cool completely, cover and refrigerate, and serve cold.

www.ingramcontent.com/pod-product-compliance
Lightning Source LLC
Chambersburg PA
CBHW050050260726
48658CB00005B/1867